Skin Cancer Therapy

The Life-Changing Routine To Permanently Prevent And Cure Skin Cancer

By

Dr. Rebecca T. Luna

INTRODUCTION

CHAPTER 1

Most Prevalent Skin Cancers

Cancer Of The Basal Cells.

Carcinoid Squamous Cells.

Melanocyte Cancer

Melanoma

Skin Cancer Signs And Symptoms

The Following Characteristics For Basal Cells Carcinoma May Be Present In Two Or More Cases:

The Following Symptoms Of Squamous Cell Carcinoma Include

Instances Of Merkel Cell Cancer Include

CHAPTER 2

Can Drawing On Yourself Cause Skin Cancer?

The Purpose Of Skin Drawing

What Distinguishes Drawing From Getting A Tattoo

How Can You Determine Whether A Tattoo Will Cause Skin Cancer

CHAPTER 3

The Risks, Factors, And Prevention

Sunburn May Be Avoided by Taking The Following Precautions

SCREENING

Information about Skin Cancer Screening For Non-melanoma

In A skin Self-examination, Do The Following Actions:

CHAPTER 4

Study Up Cancer Rehabilitation

surgery

Questions To Ask About Receiving Treatments That Include Medicines

Questions To Consider When Arranging For additional Care

CONCLUSION

INTRODUCTION

A tumor forms when healthy cells start to alter and expand out of control, which is how cancer starts. Both malignant and benign tumors may exist. A malignant tumor has cancer because it may develop and spread to other bodily areas. A benign tumor has the potential to develop but not spread.

Each year, more than 3 million Americans get a diagnosis with skin cancer, making it the most frequent kind of cancer. Early detection of skin cancer often allows for the use of topical medicines, dermatologist office treatments, or outpatient surgery as the primary forms of treatment. A physician who focuses on disorders of the skin is known as a dermatologist. Thus, fewer than 1% of cancer-related fatalities are attributable to skin cancer.

When skin cancer is further advanced, it may need to be managed by a multidisciplinary team, which often consists of a dermatologist, a surgical oncologist, a radiation oncologist, and a medical oncologist. Together, these specialists and the patient will discuss the best course of action for treating the malignancy. In rare cases, the surgical oncologist will advise having surgery done in an operating room when the cancer treatment is too involved for an office environment. Other times, the team may advise radiation therapy and/or medical therapies using pills taken orally or intravenously instead of or in addition to surgery.

CHAPTER 1

Most Prevalent Skin Cancers

Skin cancer comes in 4 primary subtypes

Cancer Of The Basal Cells.

The spherical cells in the bottom epidermis are called basal cells. These cells account for around 80% of skin malignancies. Basal cell carcinomas are the name given to these tumors. Although it may occur anywhere on the skin, basal cell carcinoma most often appears on the head and neck. The major causes of it are sun exposure and radiation treatment that was given to youngsters. Rarely does this particular kind of skin cancer migrate to other body areas and develops slowly in most cases.

Carcinoid Squamous Cells.

Flat, scale-like cells known as squamous cells make up the majority of the epidermis. Squamous cell carcinomas, which account for 20% of skin malignancies, are those that arise from these cells. Sun exposure is the primary cause of squamous cell carcinoma, which may be seen in various skin types. On skin that has been burnt, harmed by chemicals, or exposed to x-rays, it may also manifest. On the lips, at the locations of old scars, and on the skin around the mouth, anus, and vagina, squamous cell carcinoma is often seen. Between 2% and 5% of squamous cells, carcinomas disseminate to other bodily regions.

Melanocyte Cancer

A rare disease called Merkel cell cancer is very aggressive or rapidly developing. It begins in the hair follicles and in hormone-producing cells that are located immediately below the epidermis. It often affects the head and neck area.

Merkel cell cancer is also known as cutaneous neuroendocrine carcinoma. Get more information about neuroendocrine tumors.

Melanoma

Where the epidermis and dermis converge, melanocytes, a kind of cell, are dispersed. These cells generate melanin pigment, which gives skin its color. The most dangerous kind of skin cancer, melanoma, develops in melanocytes. It causes roughly 1% of all skin cancer cases.

Squamous cell carcinoma and basal cell carcinoma may sometimes be combined under the umbrella term "keratinocyte carcinoma." This is because they start in keratinocytes, a specific kind of skin cell. To separate keratinocyte carcinoma and Merkel cell cancer from melanoma, the term "non-melanoma skin cancer" is used in this manual.

The following guide does not include all non-melanoma skin cancers, including cutaneous (skin) lymphomas, Kaposi sarcoma, skin adnexal tumors, and sarcomas.

Skin Cancer Signs And Symptoms

The following signs and symptoms might be present in someone with Merkel cell, squamous cell, or basal cell carcinoma. Non-melanoma skin cancer patients may sometimes lack any of these modifications. Or, a medical disease other than cancer might be to blame for a symptom's occurrence.

The primary indicator of skin cancer is changing in the skin. It is crucial to see your doctor if you detect a change in your skin since each kind of skin cancer may manifest itself differently. The following is a list of common skin characteristics.

The Following Characteristics For Basal Cells Carcinoma May Be Present In Two Or More Cases:

•A wound that is still open after many weeks and bleeds, oozes, or crusts
•A crimson, inflamed patch or region that may crust or itch but is seldom painful.
•A bulge that is transparent, pearly white, shining, or pink, red, or pink

•A pink growth with a crusty center depression and a raised border.
•A scar-like, white, yellow, or waxy region that often has a blurry boundary

The Following Symptoms Of Squamous Cell Carcinoma Include

•Anything that resembles a wart
•A persistent, scaly red spot that may bleed freely and has erratic bordering
•An ongoing open wound for weeks
•An elevated growth with a central depression, rough skin, and rough edges

Instances Of Merkel Cell Cancer Include

Luminous, firm, and painless skin bumps These lumps may be blue, pink, or red. Some skin cancer varieties travel via the nerves. Itching, soreness, numbness, tingling, or a sensation of ants crawling beneath the skin may result from this. A lump or bulge beneath the skin in the neck, armpit, or groin may also be an indication.

Please consult with your doctor if you have any concerns about any changes you notice. Along with other things, your doctor will enquire as to how long and how often the symptoms have been bothering you. This might include the occurrence date, the duration of the skin condition, and any other symptoms you might be feeling. This process, known as diagnostic, aims to identify the root of the issue.

Most skin cancer instances may be cured by having the malignancy surgically removed or by using a topical medication. A multidisciplinary team of specialists will consult with a patient in more complex circumstances to examine various treatment options and create a strategy that has the highest possibility of curing or treating the condition.

Symptom relief will be a crucial component of cancer care and therapy, especially for advanced skin cancer. Palliative care and supportive care are two names for this. It is continued throughout therapy once it has begun. Make sure to discuss all of your symptoms, especially any new or changing symptoms, with your healthcare staff.

CHAPTER 2

Can Drawing On Yourself Cause Skin Cancer?

We reflect on ourselves throughout our lives. Until we get the outcome that pleases us, we draw using crayons, pencils, pens, and markers. We seldom lean on ourselves to impress anybody other than ourselves.

Drawing on oneself is often seen as a joyful, safe hobby, but this isn't always the case.

You've likely heard that acquiring a tan in the sun might result in skin cancer. It may surprise you to find that your preferred tattoo artist could potentially put you in danger.

Therefore, the simple answer is NO, drawing on yourself or anyplace else does not increase your risk of developing skin cancer. According to research, tattoo inks do not cause skin cancer but may contain certain particular components that may result in other issues.

The Purpose Of Skin Drawing

A few years ago, self-portrait sketching on the internet became popular. Numerous individuals now produce and share their body art online. Why, however, do they do it? At first look, it could be challenging to comprehend.

The tattoos and paintings, however, have a lot of significance, and we should make an effort to comprehend them.
We may not be seeing what we believe we are. More than simply a new social media trend is at play here. It's about discovering oneself and becoming well.

Drawing on oneself is often seen as a joyful, safe hobby, but this isn't always the case.

You've likely heard that acquiring a tan in the sun might result in skin cancer. It may surprise you to find that your preferred tattoo artist could potentially put you in danger.

What Distinguishes Drawing From Getting A Tattoo

Although both tattoos and drawings are two-dimensional works of art, there is a definite distinction between the two.

Tattoos may be seen as indelible designs that have been applied to the body. In contrast to drawings, which are made of ink and graphite, these paintings are made of pigments and dyes.

However, neither painters nor tattoo artists consider tattoos to be just a painting that has been inked into a person's flesh. They consider tattoos to be a kind of art in and of themselves.
Do you know how long it takes to get a tattoo? Tattoos are thought of as permanent works of art. It may take many hours to obtain a tattoo.
If you think about it, it is rather strange.

Drawings may be completed in as little as 30 minutes. And the reason for this is that tattoos aren't like conventional art. They are a wound that the artist must constantly fill up with color.

How Can You Determine Whether A Tattoo Will Cause Skin Cancer

You undoubtedly already know that tanning beds should be avoided. How would you proceed, however, if you were concerned that your tattoo would cause skin cancer?

Approximately 1 in 5 Americans, according to the CDC, have tattoos. Twenty percent of the tattoos were applied by unlicensed tattoo artists who did not follow proper procedures to avoid infection.

If the customer did any study before having the tattoo, many of these situations may be avoided.

While it is true that skin cancer may be brought on by exposure to the sun, certain individuals may be more at risk than others.

To fully comprehend the origins and methods of action of this complicated illness, skin cancer, much more study is still required.

You are exposed to numerous different kinds of cancer-causing substances when you get a tattoo, including certain colors and preservatives. These substances can enter your circulation and go to your lymph nodes.

The lymph nodes are a part of the immune system and include cells that assist your body in identifying and combating illness.

CHAPTER 3

The Risks, Factors, And Prevention

You may be able to lessen your chance of developing skin cancer. For additional information about your risk of cancer, speak with your medical team.

The risk of acquiring skin cancer is decreased by lowering exposure to UV radiation, especially by limiting time spent in the sun and avoiding indoor tanning. All ages should pay attention to this, but those with additional risk factors should pay particular attention. Over time, sun damage accumulates.

Sunburn May Be Avoided by Taking The Following Precautions

•Put on sun-protective apparel and a wide-brimmed hat to block the sun from your face, neck, and ears. UV protection factor (UPF)-labeled fabrics may provide superior protection in the form of clothing. Additionally advised is UV-protective eyewear.

•Use a broad-spectrum sunscreen all year long that is SPF 30 or higher that protects against UVA and UVB rays. Every two hours, or immediately after periods of intense perspiration or time spent in the water, reapply at least 1 ounce of sunscreen to your whole body.

•Steer clear of sunbathing for fun.

•Use sunlamps, tanning beds, or tanning clinics sparingly.

•Regularly check your skin. Both professional medical exams and self-examinations should be part of this. Find out more about doing a self-examination.

According to studies, those who had two or more prior cases of skin cancer and took a 500mg pill of nicotinamide, a kind of vitamin B3, twice daily had a 23% decrease in skin cancers other than melanoma. Before ingesting any supplements, see a physician.

Even while some study says that most individuals only need 15 minutes of daily contact with the sun to make adequate vitamin D, limiting your exposure to the sun may decrease your body's production of the vitamin. Patients who get little sun exposure should discuss with their doctor how to get enough vitamin D in their diet, including via the use of supplements. Your doctor may do a quick blood test to determine your vitamin D levels.

SCREENING

Before you have any symptoms or indications, screening is performed to search for cancer. Scientists have created and are still creating tests that can be used to check someone for certain forms of cancer before any symptoms or indicators show up.

The main objectives of cancer screening are:

•By detecting cancer at an earlier and more curable stage, the number of fatalities from the illness may be reduced or eliminated.

•Reduce the number of persons who develop the illness

•Find out more about the fundamentals of cancer screening.

Information about Skin Cancer Screening For Non-melanoma

Skin cancer awareness and early diagnosis are crucial. Patients or their relatives diagnose more than 75% of non-melanoma skin malignancies. Skin cancer may be found early, when the illness is more likely to be treated, by knowing the early warning symptoms and doing routine self-examinations of your skin.

Self-examinations have to be carried out in front of a full-length mirror in a room with good lighting. The scalp and back of the neck should be checked by a second person. Non-melanoma skin cancer most typically starts in areas of pale skin that are regularly exposed to the sun. Squamous cell carcinoma usually develops in less frequently exposed skin, such as the lower legs, among those with a darker complexion.

In A skin Self-examination, Do The Following Actions:

•In a mirror, check the front, rear, right, and left sides of the body while raising your arms.

•The outer and inner forearms, upper arms (particularly the difficult-to-see back area), and hands should all be carefully examined when bending the elbows.

•Examine the soles and gaps between the toes on the front, sides, and back of the legs and feet.

•To raise the hair and use a hand mirror to check the scalp and back of the neck, part of the hair.

•Use a hand mirror to examine your buttocks, back, and genitalia.

•If your barber or hairstylist has seen a worrisome lesion on your scalp or beneath your beard, or if you discover any of the following when doing a self-examination, speak with your doctor right once.

•A skin growth that displays the symptoms and telltale indications of non-melanoma skin cancer

•A fresh skin growth

•An existing mole or lesion that has undergone a strange transformation

•A wound that does not disappear after two weeks

CHAPTER 4

Study Up Cancer Rehabilitation

Based on the kind of cancer you have, your unique treatment plan, and your general health, discuss with your doctor your likelihood of experiencing these side effects. You could have certain physical exams, scans, or blood tests to help discover and manage any late effects from a therapy that is known to have certain side effects.

Maintaining a personal health record
To create a unique follow-up care plan, you and your doctor should collaborate. Discuss any worries you may have

regarding your potential physical or psychological well-being. ASCO provides documents to assist you to keep track of your cancer treatment and create a survivorship care strategy after it is over.

This is also a good moment to discuss who will oversee your follow-up treatment with your doctor. Others return to their primary doctor's care or another healthcare provider, while other survivors continue to visit a specialist such as an oncologist or dermatologist. This choice is influenced by several variables, including the kind and stage of cancer, any side effects, the insurance company's policies, and your personal preferences.

Share your cancer treatment summary and survivorship care plan forms with them, as well as with any other future healthcare providers, if a doctor who was not directly engaged in

Your follow-up care will be under the supervision of your cancer care.

The medical personnel who will look after you for the rest of your life would greatly benefit from knowing specifics about your cancer treatment.

Making choices towards a healthy lifestyle

It is crucial to take precautions to prevent future harm to your skin since many individuals who are treated for skin cancer live active, outdoor lifestyles. Exercise outside before 10:00 AM or after 4:00 PM. To prevent additional skin damage while you are outside, dress in long sleeves, slacks, broad-spectrum sunscreen, UV-protective eyewear, and a wide-brimmed hat. Find out more about preventing sun damage to your skin.

Following accepted health recommendations including quitting smoking, drinking in moderation, eating a healthy diet, and managing stress are suggested for those healing from skin cancer. Your strength and energy levels may be restored by routine physical exercise. Based on your requirements, physical capabilities, and level of fitness, your medical staff may assist you in developing an appropriate exercise program. Learn more about selecting a healthy lifestyle.

surgery

What kind of surgery am I going to have?

How much time will it take to get rid of the lesion?

How will the surgical site that results from the excision of the lesion be stitched up, fixed, or rebuilt?

What can you tell me about the surgical recuperation process? Do activities have restrictions? If yes, how long?

After the cancer is removed, will there be persistent pain? If so, what kinds of pain treatment plans, such as prescription drugs or relaxation exercises, are offered?

What kind of scar will be left after the procedure? What is the expected healing time?

If I encounter any adverse effects, who
should I speak to? When exactly?
Do this surgery's potential long-term
repercussions include anything else?

**Questions to consider before radiation
therapy**
•Which kind of radiation treatment is
advised?
•What does this therapy hope to
accomplish?
•How much time would it take to
administer this treatment?

What negative effects should I be prepared
for during treatment?

If I encounter any adverse effects, who
should I speak to? When exactly?

What potential long-term impacts may this therapy have?

What steps may be taken to minimize the negative effects?

Questions To Ask About Receiving Treatments That Include Medicines

What kind of medicine is advised?

What does this therapy hope to accomplish?

How much time would it take to administer this treatment?

Will a hospital or clinic be where I obtain this care? Will I bring it home instead?

What negative effects should I be prepared for during treatment?

If I encounter any adverse effects, who should I speak to? When exactly?

What potential long-term impacts may this therapy have?

What steps may be taken to minimize The negative effects?

Questions To Consider When Arranging For additional Care

What is the likelihood of a cancer recurrence? Should I keep an eye out for certain symptoms or signs?

What potential late effects or long-term adverse effects may my cancer therapy have?

How frequently should I be checked to look out for further skin cancers?

What more tests will I need as a result, and how frequently?

How may I get a treatment overview and a survivorship care plan for my records?

Who will be in charge of managing my aftercare?

How can I avoid developing skin cancer in the future?

What resources are accessible to me for support? To my loved ones?

CONCLUSION

The U.S. Surgeon General highlights in this Call to Action the need of taking immediate action to address the important public health issue of skin cancer. Skin cancer rates in the US have risen over the years, particularly rates of melanoma, despite attempts to reduce risk factors. 1,13-17 More than one-third of Americans say they've had a sunburn recently,226 and certain demographics often engage in indoor tanning. 132,133 To solve the public health issue of skin cancer, we must cooperate. We are aware that with sufficient funding and a coordinated strategy, community-wide, comprehensive initiatives to prevent skin cancer may be successful.

People must receive the information they need to make knowledgeable decisions about sun protection, policies must support these efforts, youth must be shielded from the dangers of indoor tanning, and adequate funding for skin cancer research and surveillance must be made if the population is to experience a decrease in skin cancers. It won't be easy to accomplish these objectives. Dedication, inventiveness, competence, and the coordinated efforts of several partners in prevention across numerous sectors will be necessary. Many of these partners are already fervently engaged, but more coordination and assistance are required to broaden the impact of their initiatives. The following actions are the plans presented in this text. To reduce the escalating rate of skin cancer in the United States, we urgently need to take action.